Breath Prayers
for
Cancer Patients

spiritual nurture for your soul

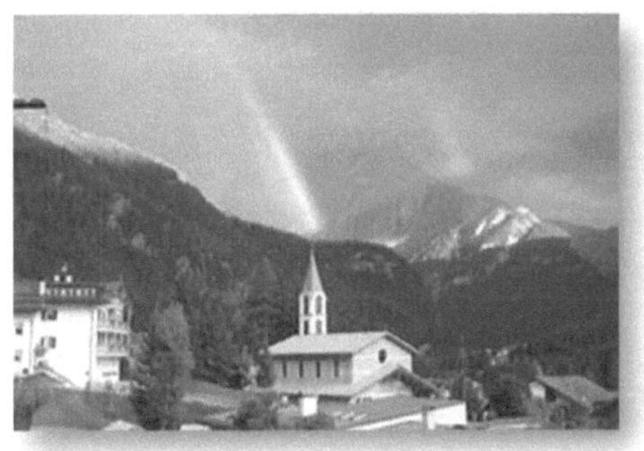

by Esther Gillie
© 2018

Table of Contents

Introduction

What are breath prayers?
*Breath prayers are short prayers, usually based on Scriptures, that help people be aware of God's presence.

*They remind the person praying of who God is and how much God cares for them.

*Breath prayers were known to the early church fathers and mothers as a way to pray without ceasing.

*They are easy–to–recall two-part phrases that are prayed in rhythm with a person's breathing.

How do breath prayers help cancer patients?
Cancer patients and people with chronic illness face many challenges that can be frightening and painful. Often they feel alone and scared.

These simple prayers can help them connect with the presence of God, encourage them, and give them strength and hope in times of distress.

Breath prayers can be prayed anywhere — in a doctor's office, surgery, an infusion center, a scanning machine or anywhere else a patient goes.

How do you pray a breath prayer?
Get as comfortable and relaxed as possible. Close your eyes if you can. Focus on your breathing. Breathe as deeply as you can. When you are ready to pray, think/pray the first part of the prayer as you inhale. Think/pray the second part of the prayer as you exhale. Throughout the book, a forward slash (/) will mark suggested places in the wording of the prayer for the inhale (before the forward slash) and exhale (after the forward slash).

Can I write my own breath prayers?
Absolutely! Once you are comfortable with this method of praying, the Holy Spirit can bring appropriate phrases to mind which address the particular situation you are facing.

May God bless you as you pray.

Breath Prayers for Spiritual Concerns

Helpful when you doubt the existence of God, when you question what God is like, if you feel that God does not care about what you are going through, when you wonder about what happens to you after you die.

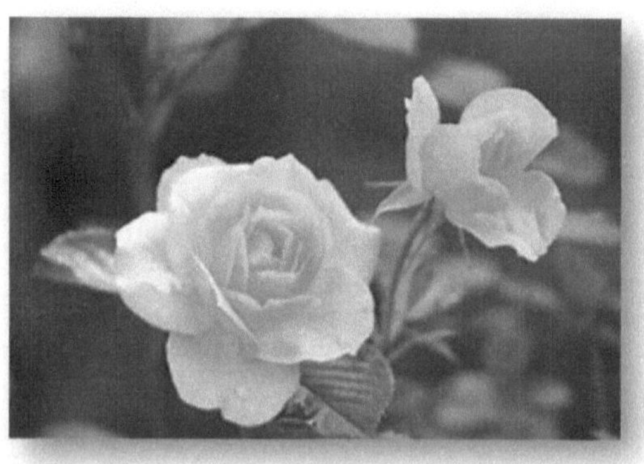

God / is

Genesis 1:1

God / is love

I John 4:8

God / is good

Psalm 34:8

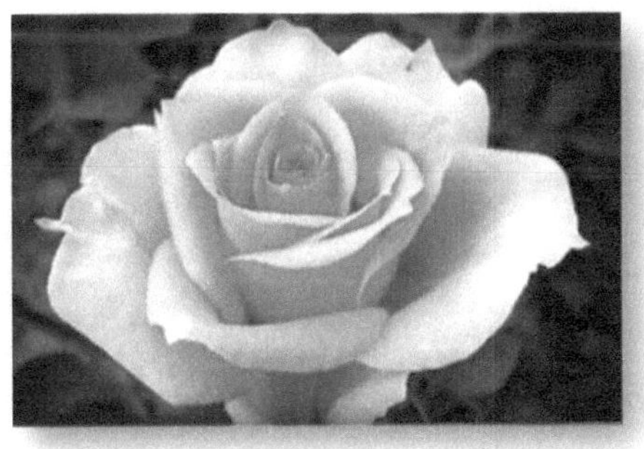

God / is light

Psalm 27:1

God is / my strength

Exodus 15:2

God is / my salvation

Psalm 27:1

God is / my refuge

Psalm 46:1

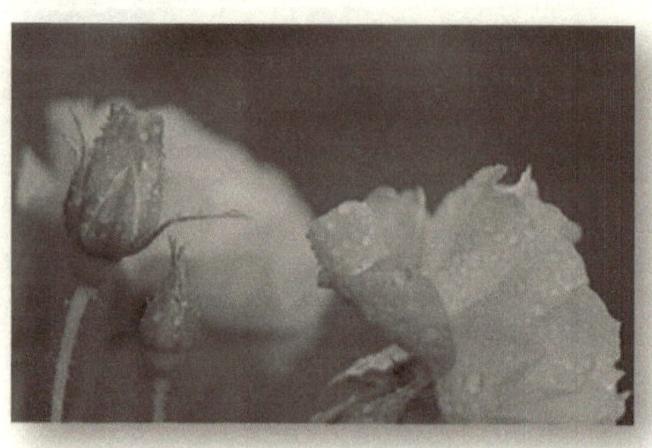

God is / my rock

Psalm 18:2

The Lord is / my Shepherd

Psalm 23:1

The Lord is / my helper

Hebrews 13:6

Jesus / loves me

John 3:16

The Lord's love / is steadfast

Psalm 103:17

Breath Prayers for Physical Concerns

Helpful before, during, and after medical tests, scans, appointments, and procedures such as chemotherapy, radiation, surgery, transplants, alternative therapies, laser treatments, and dealing with the side effects of medical interventions.

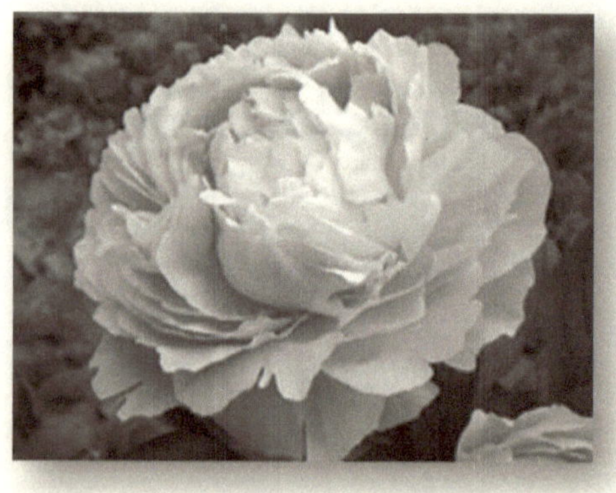

Heal me / O God

Psalm 6:2

God free me / from pain

I Chronicles 4:10

Have mercy / O Lord

Psalm 41:4

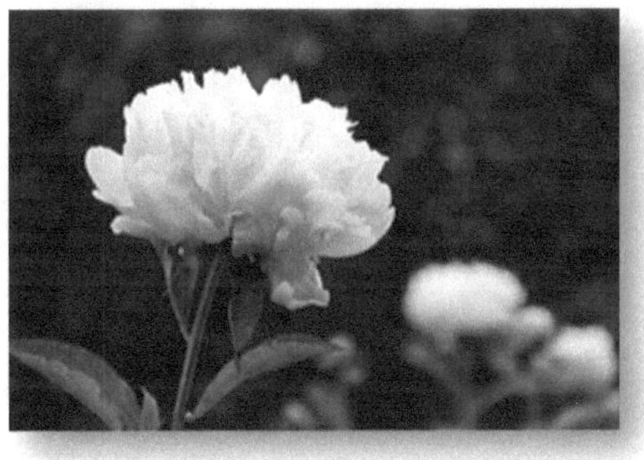

The Lord / is my strength

Psalm 22:19

God hears / my prayer

Psalm 102:1

God's word / heals me

Psalm 107:20

Restore me / O Lord

Jeremiah 33:6

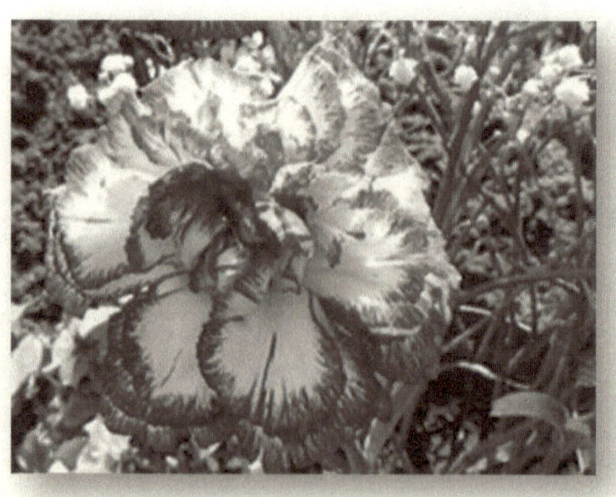

By Your wounds / I am healed

Isaiah 53:5

God heals / my disease

Psalm 103:3

Rescue me / O Lord

Psalm 33:18-19

Hear my prayer / O God

Psalm 6:9

Deliver me / O Lord

Matthew 6:13

Breath Prayers for Emotional Concerns

Helpful when you find you are afraid, anxious, angry, worried, sad, depressed, impatient, frustrated, or feel helpless.

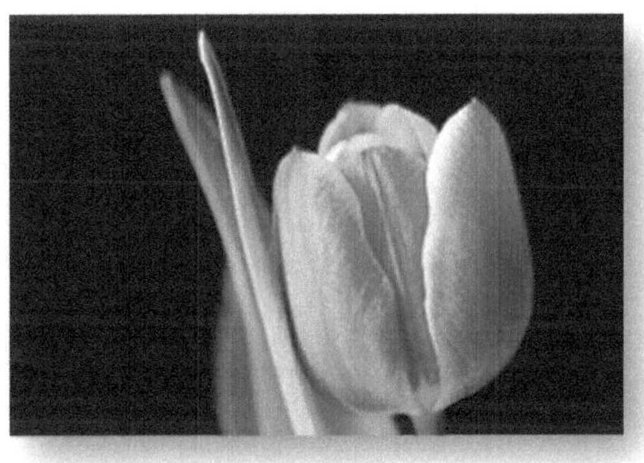

God / help me

Psalm 30:2

God's peace / upholds me

John 16:33

My times / are in God's hands

Psalm 31:15

My hope / is in God

Psalm 42:5

God has / forgiven me

I John 2:12

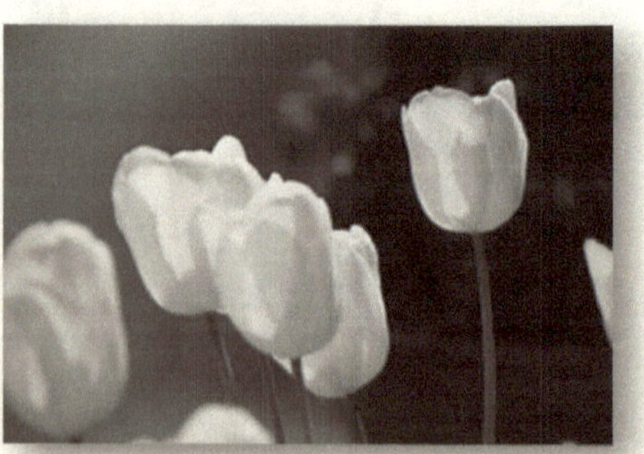

The joy of the Lord / is my strength

Nehemiah 8:10

Lord / have mercy

Psalm 4:1

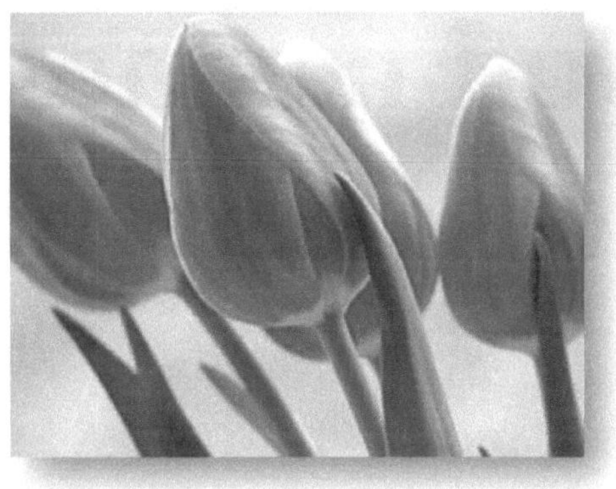

God / is with me

Psalm 46:11

Restore me / O Lord

Psalm 41:3

God / is able

2 Corinthians 9:8

God / loves me

Galatians 2:20

God has not / forsaken me

Hebrews 13:5

Breath Prayers for Social Concerns

Helpful when you feel your friends have abandoned you, when you face procedures alone, when your family and those you love live far away and cannot be with you.

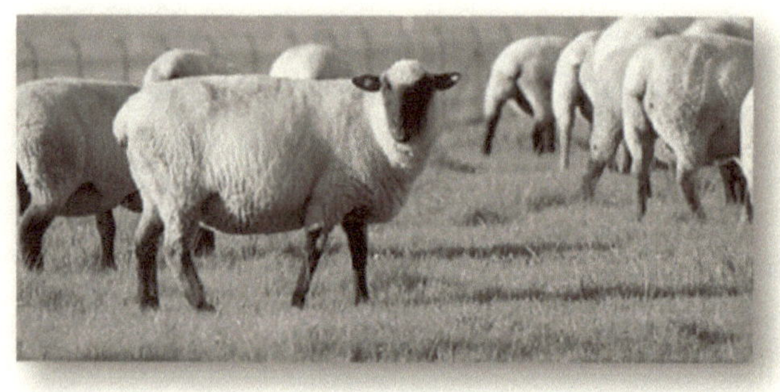

I am not alone / God is with me

John 16:32

In God alone / my soul awaits

Psalm 62:1

Be near me / Lord Jesus

Psalm 38:21

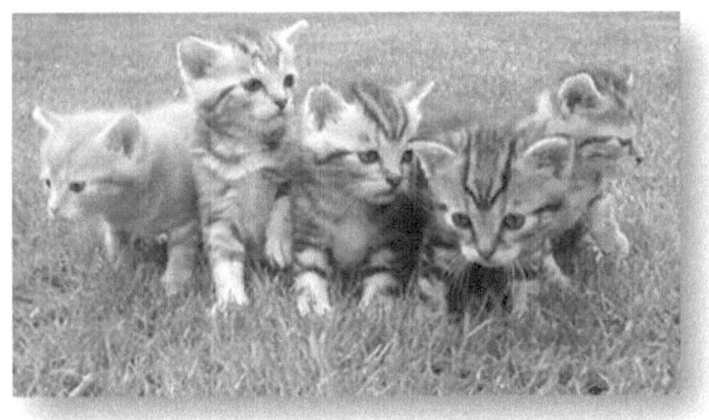

God will never / leave me

Hebrews 13:5

God will not / forsake me

Psalm 138:8

God is / with me

Isaiah 41:10

God directs / my paths

Proverbs 3:6

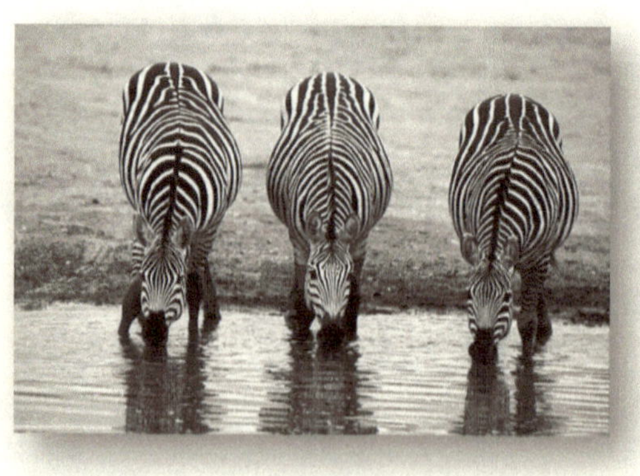

God watches / over me

Psalm 121:4

I am a member of / the body of Christ

I Corinthians 12:13

God is always / with me

Matthew 28:20

I belong / to God's family

Romans 8:16

God is closer / than a brother

Proverbs 18:24

Breath Prayers for Mental Concerns

Helpful when you experience chemo brain, find you can no longer multi-task, can't remember things you should know, have a foggy brain, or find you made mistakes balancing your checkbook.

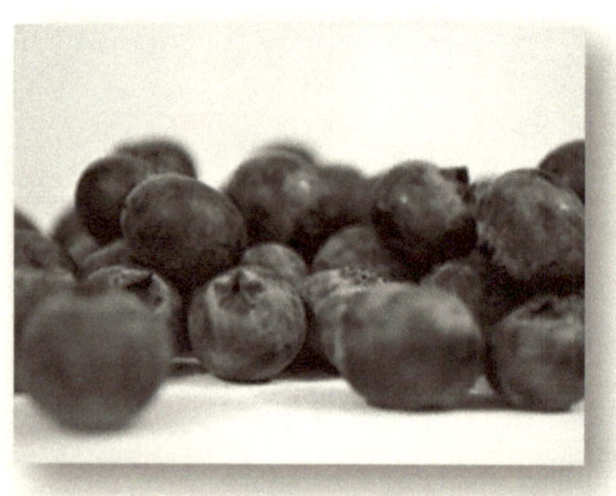

God guards / my mind

Philippians 4:7

God is / for me

Romans 8:31

The Lord / perfects me

Psalm 138:8

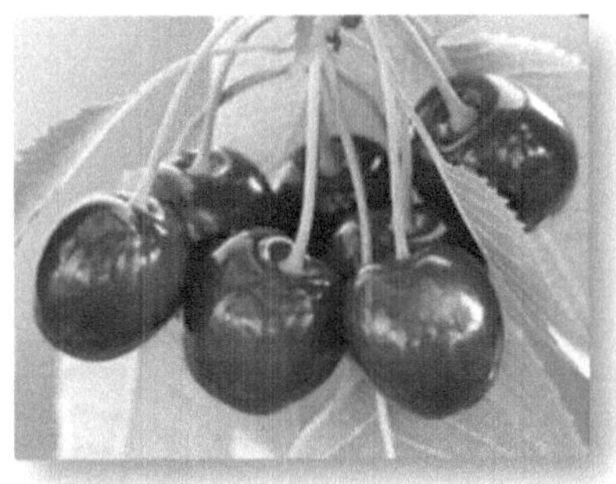

God preserves me / from trouble

Psalm 32:7

God heals me / of all afflictions

Mark 5:34

God gives me / the victory

I Corinthians 15:57

The Lord will / raise me up

James 5:15

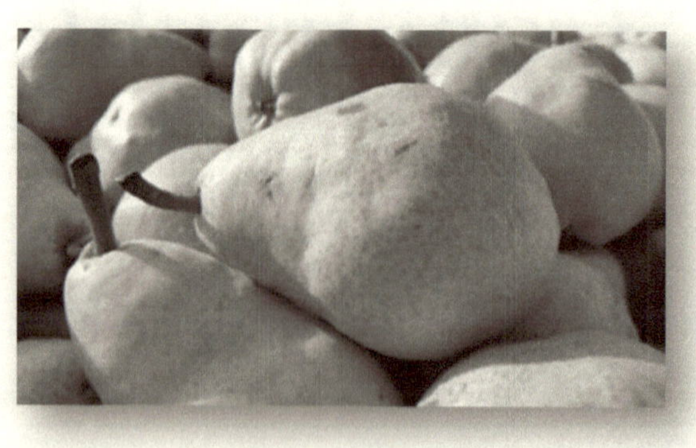

God hears / my prayers

Matthew 19:26

I have / the mind of Christ

I Corinthians 2:16

God's peace / keeps my mind clear

Philippians 4:7

I think about / God's goodness

Philippians 4:8

God will / restore me

Jeremiah 30:17

Breath Prayers for Financial Concerns

Helpful when you face a loss of income, retirement funds, a house, loss of or change in employment, or when you face expensive medical procedures or when you experience difficulties concerning health insurance.

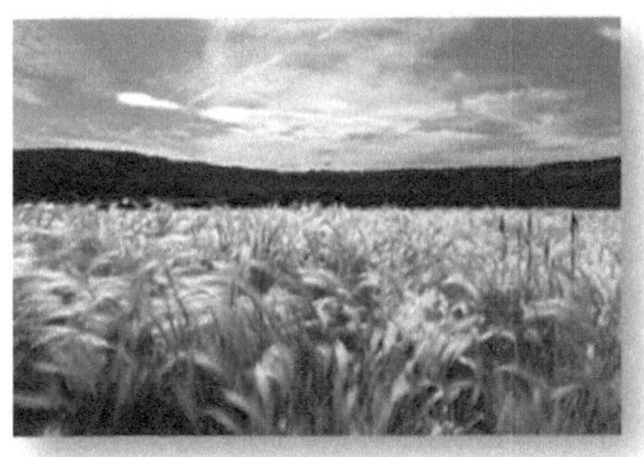

God knows / all my needs

Matthew 6:32

My God / will supply

Philippians 4:19

God is / my shelter

Psalm 61:3

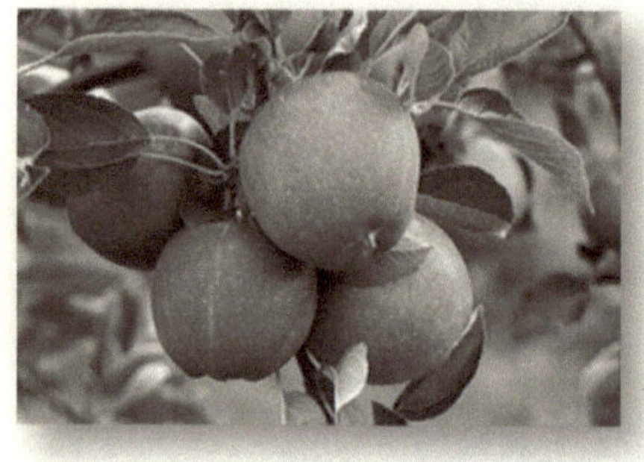

My inheritance / is forever

Psalm 37:18

I shall / not want

Psalm 23:1

God gives / good gifts

Luke 11:13

God has / blessed me

Ephesians 1:3

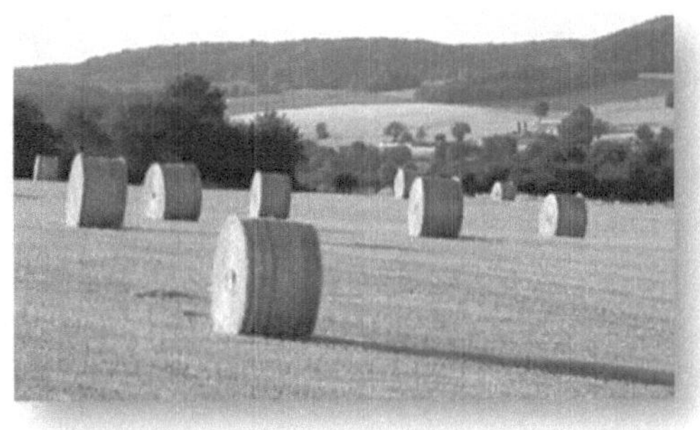

My God / is rich

Philippians 4:19

I ask the blessing /
of the Lord

I Chronicles 17:27

Be bountiful to me /
O Lord

Psalm 119:17

God is / working
things out

Romans 8:28

When I ask / I
receive

Matthew 7:8

Index of Scriptures

Genesis 1:1	Psalm 41:4
Exodus 15:2	Psalm 42:5
I Chronicles 4:10	Psalm 46:1
I Chronicles 17:27	Psalm 46:11
Nehemiah 8:10	Psalm 61:3
Psalm 4:1	Psalm 62:1
Psalm 6:2	Psalm 102:1
Psalm 6:9	Psalm 103:3
Psalm 18:2	Psalm 103:17
Psalm 22:19	Psalm 107:20
Psalm 23:1	Psalm 119:17
Psalm 27:1	Psalm 121:4
Psalm 30:2	Psalm 138:8

Psalm 31:15	Proverbs 3:6
Psalm 32:7	Proverbs 18:24
Psalm 33:7	Isaiah 41:10
Psalm 34:8	Isaiah 53:5
Psalm 37:18	Jeremiah 30:17
Psalm 38:21	Jeremiah 33:6
Psalm 41:3	Matthew 6:13

Matthew 6:32	Philippians 4:19
Matthew 7:8	Hebrews 13:5
Matthew 19:26	Hebrews 13:6
Matthew 28:20	James 5:15
Mark 5:34	I John 2:12
Luke 11:13	I John 4:8
John 3:16	Matthew 19:26
John 16:32	Matthew 28:20

John 16:33	Mark 5:34
Romans 8:16	Luke 11:13
Romans 8:28	John 3:16
Romans 8:31	John 16:32
I Corinthians 2:16	
I Corinthians 12:13	
I Corinthians 15:57	
2 Corinthians 9:8	
Galatians 2:20	
Ephesians 1:3	
Philippians 4:7	
Philippians 4:8	

Index of Breath Prayers

Be bountiful to me / O Lord
Be near me / Lord Jesus
By your wounds / I am healed
Deliver me / O Lord
God directs / my paths
God free me / from pain
God gives / good gifts
God gives me / the victory
God guards / my mind
God has / blessed me
God has / forgiven me
God has not / forsaken me
God heals / my disease

God heals me / of all afflictions
God hears / my prayer
God hears / my prayers
God / help me
God / is
God / is able
God is always / with me
God is closer / than a brother
God is / for me
God / is good
God / is light
God / is love
God is / my refuge
God is / my rock
God is / my salvation

| God is / my shelter |
| God is / my strength |
| God is / with me |
| God is / working things out |
| God knows / all my needs |
| God / loves me |
| God preserves me / from trouble |

| God watches / over me |
| God will never / leave me |
| God will not / forsake me |
| God will / restore me |
| God's peace / keeps my mind clear |
| God's peace / upholds me |
| God's Word / heals me |
| Have mercy / O Lord |

Heal me / O God
Hear my prayer / O God
I am a member of / the body of Christ
I am not alone / God is with me
I ask the blessing / of the Lord
I belong / to God's family
I have / the mind of Christ
I shall / not want
I think about / God's goodness
In God alone / my soul awaits
Jesus / loves me
Lord / have mercy
My God / is rich
My God / will supply
My hope / is in God

My inheritance / is forever
My times / are in God's hands
Rescue me / O Lord
Restore me / O Lord
The Lord / perfects me
The Lord is / my helper
The Lord is / my Shepherd
The Lord will / raise me up
The Lord's love / is steadfast
The joy of the Lord / is my strength
The Lord / is my strength
When I ask / I receive